MASSAGE

MASSAGE

✦

More Than A Technique

*A book of something to think about when pursuing
the field of massage therapy.*

Carly M. Stevenson

iUniverse, Inc.
New York Lincoln Shanghai

MASSAGE
More Than A Technique

Copyright © 2006 by Carly M. Stevenson

iUniverse books may be ordered through booksellers or by contacting:

iUniverse
2021 Pine Lake Road, Suite 100
Lincoln, NE 68512
www.iuniverse.com
1-800-Authors (1-800-288-4677)

This book is written for the person who is in the midst of changing careers and is captivated by the essence of being fulfilled in the field of massage therapy.

ISBN-13: 978-0-595-38983-4 (pbk)
ISBN-13: 978-0-595-83365-8 (ebk)
ISBN-10: 0-595-38983-X (pbk)
ISBN-10: 0-595-83365-9 (ebk)

Printed in the United States of America

A thought to ponder:

Begin each day by making a difference.
For making a difference
is truly what it's all about.

Contents

Acknowledgment

I would like to take this opportunity to thank my family and friends and the instructors I met along the way who have supported me through this challenging career change. I would like to also thank the many people who have touched my life and made a difference in it. Not only have they inspired me to be who I am, but they believe in me and also in the gift of touch I possess. Words can not express the love that I have for all of you. For me "Making a Difference is what it's all about."

A thought to ponder:

Live for today, dream for tomorrow and plan for the future.

What Brings You Here

Welcome! What brings you here to consider becoming a Massage Therapist? Have you been in search of a career that provides stability for your family? Are your friends or family encouraging you to pursue a life long dream, or is it the fact that you want to help people feel good not only on the outside but on the inside as well? Could it be that you have just spent a day at the spa and you are captivated by the sheer essence of feeling relaxed and rejuvenated (this is how I became a massage therapist)? Whatever the case may be, this challenging career opportunity awaits you, and now what do you do?

It is never easy to start a new career, **nor** is it too late. You may consider job shadowing a Massage Therapist for a day to see what his/her day entails. Remember that no two days will be the same; however, it can help shed a little light on the subject. This is also a great way to obtain information upfront and get answers from a person in the field.

Here are a handful of questions and areas of interest to uncover when preparing for a career in the Massage Therapy field:

- Educate yourself with information pertaining to the field of massage.
- What type of schooling/education is needed?
- Where can you find a massage school in your local area?
- Gather information on several different programs to see which one fits not only your current life style but your goals and needs as well.
- Become familiar with the different organizations for Massage Therapy; AMTA (American Massage Therapy Association), NCBTMB(National Certification Board for Therapeutic Massage and Body work)
- Do you have what it takes to succeed as a Massage Therapist?
- Where will you find work?
- Will the pay be adequate for your needs?

A thought to ponder:

**The decisions we make today will become our tomorrow
without even trying.**

My Mission and Vision

The purpose behind publishing this book was to not only gain more insight for myself, but to provide information to help others who are considering a challenging career change into the massage therapy field.

I have not always been a person who has set goals and achieved them or a person who strived to do well. Once I realized the importance in succeeding, I then decided to put forth all my effort in everything I do. My clients say they "feel my passion" for the profession of massage therapy, and that is so wonderful to hear.

I had decided that without exposing certain aspects of myself I would not be able to grow. I have written out my mission and vision statement. I was exposed to this type of training prior to becoming a massage therapist. This has helped me recognize the type of person I want to be and has given me the courage and strength to move forward.

The mission and vision statement that I have written for myself reveals the type of person I am and how I present myself as a Certified Massage Therapist. I would like to take this opportunity to share both my mission and vision statements with you.

MISSION STATEMENT

My Clients Come First.

As a Massage Therapist, it is not only my duty but also my responsibility to treat my clients with the utmost respect and integrity they are so deserving of. I need to provide not only a safe, clean environment but also an environment that creates an atmosphere of security and serenity for my clients. I am responsible for their personal well being, while performing any type of bodywork and/or treatment. Though I cannot and will not diagnose any diseases for my clients, it is my responsibility to refer my clients to the proper Health Care Professionals if I see, feel, or sense a health issue.

VISION STATEMENT
"MAKING A DIFFERENCE IS WHAT IT'S ALL ABOUT"

Yes, I know what you are thinking. What a short vision. But you see making a **difference** is what it's all about. Nothing more-nothing less.

As you begin the journey into a new, exciting, and challenging career stop and take a moment to discover what it is that you want to do with it.

Use the space provided to jot down some ideas of what you want your clients to say about you as a massage therapist.

- Do I work for someone or for myself?
- How do you get your name out there?
- What about the registration and licensing?
- What kind of insurance is needed?
- What about after graduation, what is expected from a schooling stand point?

These are just a few questions on the endless list that will run through your mind as you begin to **explore** your own ability to become a Massage Therapist and the nature of the field.

STOP RIGHT THERE!!! We all have dreams and desires. You are the only one to make those dreams and desires a reality. So do what feels right and follow your heart. Do you want to wake up someday and say "what if???" I know I didn't.

Use the space below to jot down any additional questions you may have.

A thought to ponder:

Be captivated by who you are.
Your integrity will pave the way to success.

Where to Begin When Getting Started

CONGRATULATIONS! You have decided to pursue a career in the field of Massage Therapy. GREAT!! Now what? First you will need to find a school. The internet is a great source and can provide a wealth of information. If you do not have access to the internet, the public library or the local book store would also be a great source of information.

Depending on your location, each city and state has a set of regulations and requirements that need to be met in order for a person to be registered as a Massage Therapist. It is always a great idea to gain as much information as possible on the front end so there are no hidden surprises that have not been accounted for.

First, find the school location nearest you and see what requirements need to be met **prior to registration**. Next, here are a few questions to ask upfront:

- What are the required courses needed to become eligible for certification?

- What is the time frame of school, and is there an active syllabus for review?

- How many students are allowed to register per graduating class?

- Is there a way of assisting the school after graduation for the training of other massage therapists?

- What cost is associated with tuition and what cost are **EXTRA**? (Remember no hidden surprises)?

- What is the school's success rate and does the school assist in job placement upon completion?

- What is the grading system? Is it a strict pass or fail or is each class graded individually?

- What is required after certification to retain the title of Massage Therapist?

I am sure you will think of a few more questions that I have not provided. Write them down, and make sure you are clear on what the expectations are so there are no hidden surprises once you are signed up for class and are ready to go.

Use the space below to jot down any additional questions you may have.

A thought to ponder:

Treat each client like gold, for they hold the key to your success.

The Gift of Touch and the Power Behind It

All of us have a certain aura about ourselves. Whether it's how we look, walk, speak, dress, think, interact with others or present ourselves, we are all different.

This is very true with massage therapists as well. In the world of massage therapy, the "gift of touch" possessed is different as well for all Massage Therapists. There are no two alike, even though the same techniques are taught around the world.

Their style of touch is a "gift", not a lesson learned. Each massage therapist presents his/her own style, and his/her own technique that he/she has learned and perfected. His/her touch can convey a story so to speak. You, as a massage therapist, must be cognizant of the fact that your clients will be able to tell if the work you are doing flows, if you enjoy being there or if there is a sense of reservation in your touch.

Based on the approach you take as a massage therapist, your clients will know if you truly want to be there (giving a massage) or not. The passion and desire that comes from being a massage therapist will show through the work you do. I have heard people say 'the massage therapist I saw for my last appointment seemed to be in a robotic state.' I have heard other people say 'I love my therapist!!'

While some massage therapists have a firm or strong touch, others will possess a passive yet softer touch. If you're like some massage therapists, the client can feel the energy from within you; the hand pressure and techniques used have a way of creating a warm connected or inviting feeling for the client which is incredible.

Always remember that the difference in touch lies in the perception of the recipient. In general, we all need to remember that perception is reality whether we like to admit it or not. You will find that everyone you work with will have a different perception of you as a therapist. Good or bad the client is the determining factor of how the massage is going. Each client's tolerance or threshold for pressure and sensory touch will be different, and the expectation of what feels good and what does not will be different as well. So remember to check in with your client for the amount of pressure you are using. We as massage therapists do not want to hurt anyone.

Another aspect to remember is that Massage Therapists are very unique in their own special way and have a way about them that promotes health and well being. They make people feel good, not only on the inside but the outside as well. Always remember that if your hands feel cold to you, they will probably feel really cold to your client. I have had my clients tell me that my hands feel very therapeutic to them. This is great feedback for a therapist to hear.

Do not fret that your touch is not worthy for others to experience. Be proud of who you are and the gift of touch you have to offer. As I said before, the perception lies within the recipient. Some clients out there will enjoy the gift of touch you have to offer.

A thought to ponder:

**The impossible can be achieved
only if you try.**

Aligning Your Goals and Finding A Niche

The field of Massage Therapy is ever growing. New talents are exploding from schools around the world. As I mentioned before, the same techniques are being taught everywhere, but homing in on a specific niche and setting realistic goals will not only help you succeed, but will set you apart from the competition.

The key to being successful is finding a niche and staying with it. Differentiate yourself from the rest. Provide services and information that is not only different from that of other massage therapists but beneficial as well.

Goal setting is also very important to being successful. **Jot down your ideas of what, where, and when** you would like to accomplish the goals you have set. Talk about your goals. Share your goals with others and/or find a mentor to help guide you. Get out there and speak with massage therapist already doing the job. Define what you would like to achieve with the skills you will have. The more realistic the goal the less chance there is for you to become frustrated. Never give up!!

Finding a niche in the marketplace is easier said than done. An array of opportunities exist out there, even one that fits your needs and the needs of the client base that you are striving to create. These questions have to be answered, prior to selecting a direction or target market.

Here are a few examples of what type of service you could provide to your potential client base:

- Sports Massage—align yourself with sporting events or fitness centers.
- Therapeutic Massage—direct your skills toward a Chiropractic office.
- Geriatrics—reach the elderly in a hospice or nursing home environment.

- On-Site Chair Massage at Corporations—and target the stressful work arena.
- Relaxation, in a Spa or Salon setting.

Again, once you decide the direction and then align your goals, it will be easier to find a niche in the field of massage.

Once you have decided the direction you want to approach, then you need to pick the setting for your business. Opportunities are endless for business settings, ranging from your home to the airport. Make sure the area you want to target is in-line with the setting for practice.

Also when working with your clients, tailor their session around the type of service they are looking for and what you offer. Is the client here for relaxation or some sort of treatment? Is the client a professional athlete and looking to enhance performance? Or is the client looking for the only cosmetic aspect. These are very important aspects of questioning which will assist you in selecting your niche.

Use the space below to jot down some notes as they come to mind.

A thought to ponder:

As NASA has sent our astronauts to reach for the stars, do the same.

Opportunities Are Endless For Employment—Be Creative

By now you're probably wondering where you could possibly obtain employment. The list is endless. Once again begin by deciding on the type of client you want to work with, then pick a setting that complements the client base.

Here are a variety of settings available to you as a therapist:

Medical Setting

- Hospital
- Chiropractic Office
- Dentist Office
- Doctor Office
- Assisted Living Facilities

Recreational Setting

- Shopping Mall
- Salon/Spa
- Massage Office
- Group Practice
- Fitness Club
- Golf Course
- In Home Spa

Travel Setting

- Airport

- Resort/Hotel

- Cruise Ship

- Bed and Breakfast

Professional Setting

- Corporation

- Insurance Company

- Law/Attorney Office

Be creative. I cannot stress enough the point that **the setting needs to fall in line with the market you intend to target.** The local phone book is a great way to find listings for various organizations that could fit the client base you have chosen. Also research the internet, if available to you, for further information. The library can also provide an array of information in finding settings or creating ideas for employment.

A thought to ponder:

Let your creativity introduce who you are.

Marketing Tools For Success—Networking With Others

Now it is time to move forward with the marketing aspect of the job. The marketing tools you chose will help pave the way in building a successful massage business.

Hopefully during your schooling for massage therapy your instructors will touch base on this subject. Marketing is much more than a simple business card and a sign or place of employment.

First of all when you're asked to think out of the box, what comes to mind? What ideas run through your head? **Never hesitate to jot down your ideas**. Keep a pen and paper handy and modify your ideas as needed. Seeing your ideas on paper will help in stimulating new ones. Jotting down your ideas will have a networking effect with the ones you have already written down.

When I am in the process of marketing I like to imagine the uniqueness of an opportunity. What ideas can and will separate me from the rest? Some of the ideas that I jot down seem a little far fetched, or not realistic while others are right on track. I also share my ideas with others and look for any hidden responses not verbally communicated. Most people you speak with will want to add their thoughts as well. Invite them to. This is also a way of gaining new view points that can assist you in making decisions.

If you chose to be open and communicate your ideas, find someone you know who will be honest with you and give you the valuable feedback you are looking for. Also be ready to hear things you might not want to hear.

Some basic approaches will aid in building you a successful business and client base. First, by deciding which direction you are headed in, you can tailor your marketing plan toward the market you have chosen.

Many tools exist that you can use to help get your name out there. Remember that advantages and disadvantages always exist to every type of marketing tool you use. Some will be more advantageous than others. You will need to try them to see what is appropriate for your business. Below are just a few to help you get started. **Remember to think outside the box.**

Verbal Communication

Word of mouth—Look at having your clients promote you. They are a great source of information. Whenever they speak of their massage they will be mentioning your name and advertising you as a therapist. Now if your clients love the work you do, HURRAY! If they do not like the work you do, OH NO! I hope that this is not a deterrent but it could be.

Seminars—Seminars allow the opportunity for you not only to promote the massage profession, but also to promote yourself. You can even offer demonstrations to show the type of work you do as a massage therapist.

Wellness programs for companies—Get in contact with the person who is in charge of the wellness program for the company to see if you can be a guest speaker, to promote you and your business.

Written Communication

Signs and fliers—Signs and billboards can get a little on the pricey side. But with some creativity you can create your own signs to help promote yourself. If you are located in a fitness center or any type of open environment, use the portable easels that many of them have. They are easy to use and you can change your information on a regular basis. Hang up fliers if able at the local grocery store or Laundromat. Also check with the local gas stations, movie theaters, dry cleaners and eateries. Anywhere there are heavy traffic areas.

Menu and Brochures of Services You Provide—I like to keep a pricelist/menu handy with me at all times to share with new potential prospects. This is a great marketing tool. Make sure it provides your name, phone number, and the hours you are available along with a description of the services you provide.

The Conveniency of Gift Certificates—Gift Certificates will become your friend. They are a great way to sell your services upfront and help those who are not sure what to purchase for that special someone.

Newspaper Article—Write an article for the local bulletin or newspaper chain. Check to see if they would be willing to designate a column to the massage profession on a weekly or monthly basis. It never hurts to check. Run a special in the Sunday newspaper as well for upcoming holidays.

Coupons and Newsletters—Advertise to your clients when you are running specials. A news letter update is a great way to communicate what is going on. Also keep your client base updated if there is a change coming in the near future such as new location or business hours.

Community Events

Special Events—Many times there are sporting or community events happening in your neck of the woods. Take the opportunity to gain exposure by supporting these types of events. Church outings and picnics are also a great way to gain exposure.

Here are also a couple of ideas that you can create with very little cost invested:

- Gift Bags—Special treatments for foot or hand services
- Trial Samples—Aromatherapy sugar or salt scrubs for the body
- Dollar Off Coupons—Offer five dollars off your next visit coupons
- Birthday Specials—Remembering your clients' birthdays.
- Referral Discounts—Always remember to take the time to thank the ones who help support you by offering a referral discount. This works great and is appreciated by your client who is promoting you as a massage therapist.
- Monthly Specials that correspond with your menu.

Payment Plans

Payment—Payment plans can range from credit card, cash or check. Payment plans can also be established in advance for a certain number of treatments based on minutes (i.e. client only wants a 40 minute massage, cost is based per minute. $40.00 is the cost for that particular massage).

Remember that the cost of your service is up to you if you choose to be an independent contractor. If you choose to be an employee, the amount of pay is driven by the establishment of employment. Some negotiating can be reached, depending upon the status of the massage therapist.

Networking is also a great way to gain referrals and stimulate your business growth. I choose to network with people who are motivated, self-driven individuals and persons of interest who are aware of the services that I provide. I happened to be at a local store and struck up a conversation with a woman with whom I worked for at a local bed and breakfast for a short period of time. How amazing is that?

No matter what, I am always thinking of how I can differentiate myself from the rest. It does not have to become this expensive adventure; however, do be clever.

A thought to ponder:

Be grateful for what you receive,
no one owes you anything.

The Never Ending Prospecting List

When you hear the word prospecting what comes to your mind? Do you struggle with where to begin? Do you wonder who could or would be a potential client? Do you get a nervous feeling in the pit of your stomach?

If there were a way to make prospecting easier, I am sure that anyone in a business that requires them to prospect would take the opportunity to do just that. But prospecting can be hard work. I know from my own experience that I have to be in the **right mood**. The happy-go-lucky, mood that is.

The reason being for the happy-go-lucky, mood is that the word "no" can have an enormous impact on you and your day. For myself I feel the happy-go-lucky mood can make prospecting a little easier to digest.

I do prospecting by phone for potential on-site chair massage business and the development of a wellness program at local companies. This allows me to get in the door and to gain potential clients outside of the company environment as well.

The first thing I do is set aside a day of the week and time for prospecting. I find that first thing in the morning works best for me. I am an early riser, so the sooner I can get a jump on prospecting the sooner my day is ready for some more exciting opportunities.

I then begin to look at the type of clients I am targeting. This is why it is important to know the client base you are targeting. I then research the phone book and internet fully. I look for markets that can help capitalize my client base and make it grow.

I proceed with a list of potential clients or establishments listing their name, phone number and address. I make sure to leave enough space to write down any pertinent information pertaining to the call. To ensure I have not created duplicate contact lists I keep all cold call lists for future reference.

Next is the big step in making the cold call. A few deep breaths will help you clear your mind and set the stage. **Remember, the contact is not able to see you, but your voice is the first impression they hear. Make it a clear, concise and a pleasant one.**

I always introduce myself, and ask to speak with the person in Human Resources or the person in charge of introducing a wellness program in the establishment. (The receptionist generally questions what the call pertains to.) I give a brief description of who I am and what I do. The receptionist then connects me to the appropriate person. I then ask if they are currently working on implementing a wellness program for their employees. I let them know what I can offer as a stress relief program and ask if they would like for me to send information in the mail to them. This allows them time for questions and allows me time to promote the benefits up front and to describe how the program can work.

Depending on the time of year when calling can make or break potential business. Companies are very busy with updating enrollment plans for new insurance benefits, hiring for the summer, reorganizing internal employees, and bringing on board new computer systems. And with companies downsizing there is little time for waste. The possibility also exist that the company is not interested at all. Always thank the person for his/her time. This is very important as well.

Try not to get discouraged. If the contact person is not interested at this time, offer to send out information for the future. Remember to also highlight the ones that ask for a call back later down the road.

Prospecting is a great way to promote you and your business. Don't let the word No stop you from pursuing new business opportunities.

A thought to ponder:

Never hesitate to be more than what is expected.

Continuing Education

Study, study, study is probably the most common phrase you will hear while in school. Even when you are out of school it will be there to keep you on track. **Education after graduation will be part of your life as long as you are a massage therapist.**

Each state has its own regulations and requirements for maintaining certification as a massage therapist. Make sure you know what the guidelines are if any, that need to be followed, after you graduate from school.

Continuing Education is a great way to separate you from the competition. Learning more about the profession of massage therapy will help you not only gain more insight, but also keep you in tune with new modalities and interest points that come into play. Focus on classes that will not only enhance your skills, but expose you to different techniques. If in doubt about what classes would best fit in your line of business, check with the school you attended for assistance.

Always keep in mind that there will be clients that have been exposed to other types of massage. If they are a regular client for you, you may consider learning the type of treatment or course of action they have been exposed to.

You will also receive mailings on classes that are being held around the country. This information is helpful in finding a location near you. You can also browse the internet for online information about upcoming events. Each class or seminar is worth a different CEU value or points. If at all possible find a person in the field and ask questions. I would hate to see you invest in a program that is not what you thought it would be.

The costs of the programs vary differently. Remember to include travel time, delays, and other expenses that are not part of the schooling/program cost when deciding what seminar or class to attend. Also make sure you can attend the number of days required for the class or seminar in order to receive full credit. You would hate to have to miss a day, spend the money and receive no CEU's.

A thought to ponder:

The greatest gifts you have are those that are shared with others.

Listen to the Client—What Did They Really Say

Hear we go. Oh, that is here we go. Sorry. I got a little carried away with hear of the ear vs. here we are. But it's true, no matter what profession you are in, your listening skills are **essential**!!! The verbal and non-verbal communication that takes place between you and your client is crucial in keeping your relationship alive.

During the massage sessions always remember, your clients will communicate signs and signals to you whether they are clear and precise or not so obvious. If the client has chosen to take the time and bring to your attention an area of concern, you, as a massage therapist, need to respond accordingly. Listen with intent and empathy. Repeat back what was said to show for one thing that you are listening but also to fully understand what the client is hoping to gain from the massage session you are about to provide.

On the other hand, beware, your clients will not always communicate with you what they are truly feeling. You may ask if the pressure is fine and they will say "yes." However, the next time they come in they could request more/less pressure from you. At the end of the session they may say "that was great" when asked how the massage was and tell a friend that the massage they received was not what they were looking for. This can be damaging to you and your business as a massage therapist.

If during a session, the client is in a non-talkative mood that could mean they have come to relax and do not want to be disturbed. Allow the clients to lead to assist you when it comes to verbal and non-verbal communication.

Along with the tone of your client's voice, his/her body language will also convey how he/she is really feeling. Not only listen with your ears but with your eyes as well. If their toes curl, the pressure of the massage could be too much or they may be ticklish. If their body seems to tense up during the massage the pressure could be too much as well.

I find it very helpful to walk my client through the service that they have selected. Remember no hidden surprises. This allows the opportunity for a discussion to take place and you have opened the door for good communication. If the client states "I do not like my feet touched," then **do not touch**. Do however make a mental note, but also place that information on the Health History Form for the next visit.

A Health History Form supplies pertinent information about your clients' medical history prior to performing any type of massage or bodywork. This form is requirement in the massage therapy field. The massage therapist is responsible for not only maintaining, but updating the form as needed.

I find also that my clients will mention different scents that they may or may not find appealing. Write it down. They may even mention the type of music they prefer to listen to or the room temperature may be too warm or too cool. Some of your clients will ask if you are using a lotion or oil. Always have both on hand, to accommodate your client. Make a mental note as well, then write it down on the Health History Form to help you prepare better for their next visit.

Listening is more than hearing with the ear. Listening involves observing your clients reactions with your eyes during the massage session. The importance of utilizing the skill of listening, **can and will** assist in making or breaking a client. Remember, we all like to be heard. Listen to your client as you would want to be listened to.

A thought to ponder:

**Rewards are endless
for those who never give up.**

The Rewards Are Endless—A Little Faith Goes A Long Way

You ask what the rewards are of being a massage therapist. Is it monetary? It is the freedom to be your own boss? Could it be the fact that you meet so many different people from so many different backgrounds? How about the many new job opportunities based on the massage session you provided for a happy client? What about making a difference in someone's life, is that considered a reward to you? Or maybe it's when your first time client rebooks with you based on the job you did.

I can only speak for myself. **I truly enjoy making a difference in someone's life.** I get this burning excitement inside when my client feels great after a massage session is over. I guess you could call it an instant gratification; a self-awareness, that is at times a little over whelming. A client's words of kindness and appreciation have more value than any amount of money, they are priceless.

The rewards for being a massage therapist are endless based on what you make of them. Approach this career with an open mind and heart. Look for the unexpected, seek to be the best you can be and the rewards will be endless. **Treat your clients like gold for they hold the key to your success**. They will be the ones who bring new clients to you or keep potential clients at bay if they did not like the service you have provided. They will also be the ones that are rebooking on a regular basis.

A little faith and patience goes a long way as well. Believe in yourself as your clients do. Others, including your clients, can see and feel the confidence you have by the way you present yourself. **As the old saying goes "a first impression" is everything**. You need to not only know, but believe as well that the skills you possess can and will make a difference in someone's life. Keep believing in yourself that you will be a great massage therapist and good things will come.

Also never be afraid to seek guidance, ask questions or simply look for support from family and friends. We all at some point and time need not only the reassurance that we will succeed, but a little pick-me-upper. Asking for help does not mean you are a failure, it helps stimulate more ideas for bigger and better opportunities.

Be thankful for the business you do receive. Your business will take time to grow and will not happen over night, try not to get discouraged. **Always remember to thank each person that refers a new client your way.** For me, the best compliment is a referral and as a therapist we can all use some of those.

Remember as well that rewards are two sided, so reward the clients that are golden to you. Provide a token of appreciation such as a free half hour birthday massage or even a homemade salt glow or sugar scrub. Your clients will appreciate your thoughtfulness.

A thought to ponder:

Fight the tide with tenaciousness.

When The Going Gets Tough—Did You Make the Right Decision?

What do you do when the going gets tough? Do you quit and give up, or do you become aggressive and fight for what you want and believe in? You can approach the not so easy road ahead with tenaciousness or let a not so pleasant day be your failing factor.

At times the massage field can be a bit overwhelming. Massage Therapy is a growing industry and the competition can be stiff. There will be days that seem less than appealing and times you will question if the skills you possess will carry you through. There will be days when you question if the decision of becoming a massage therapist is the right choice for you.

Deciding if you made the right decision is up to you. You are the only one who can determine this. You must believe in yourself before others will. The old saying goes take the bull by the horns and run with it does hold true in this field as well.

Sit back once and think what if every doctor, lawyer, hair dresser, nail technician, chiropractor, plumber, electrician and the many other professions said 'forget it.' Where would they be??? The world would have a minimal of participants in these careers and the existing ones would be overloaded.

There are a few things you can do when the going does get tough. For instance, you can be creative and send out birthday coupons to your repeat clients for $5.00 off their next visit. This will spark an interest to your client to treat themselves and also promote your business as well.

Create update newsletters. Let your clients know what is new in the world of massage and what you are doing to stay current and remain an active participant in your field. This will let your clients know that you care about what you are doing and that you want to grow in the profession of massage therapy.

Purchase a motivational book and look for ways to help improve your outlook on the positive side. Attend seminars during your down time to learn new marketing techniques, or even attend a class on sales and marketing. Look into other areas that will help enhance your profession in the massage field.

There are so many things you can do when the going gets tough to help you through the not so pleasant times. Staying positive is not the easiest, but it can help you through a tough time when you need it.

I have found that talking with a good friend, another massage therapist or mentor helps just as well. It allows you to get a different perspective and find solutions to difficulties you may encounter.

A thought to ponder:

Let your dreams be bigger than life.

A Day In the Life of A Massage Therapist

Have you begun to wonder what a day in the life of a massage therapist would be like? Have you seen someone you know as a massage therapist manage their day-to-day business and wonder how they do it? Being your own boss, is it as exciting as it looks or some make it sound?

I thought it would be interesting to share a few of my typical or not so typical days as a massage therapist. No two days will be the same. That can be good and bad, depending on how you view it. Remember the glass can be half empty or the glass can be half full…you decide.

There will be days when you will have cancellations or even no show-no call. It is easier said than done to not get upset. You feel your time is valuable, and that when there are no shows or no calls people are not respecting your time. I do travel quite a bit, and have run into this from time to time. It can and does get frustrating at times.

There will be days when you are booked every hour on the hour, and can't seem to find time to eat, drink or even take a small break. Whatever your day brings, approach it with an open mind. Find the good in the day and make it your best.

I try to utilize my time to the best of my ability depending on where I am at the time and what materials I have with me. I may spend time prospecting or working on marketing material. I create all my own advertisements and coupons, and some of my own gift certificates. I also have created a menu of services that I provide. So I may focus on this if nothing else. Or I may also be working on some CEU's and need to be studying.

I thought back to when I first started out as a massage therapist. I remember I was so proud of myself to have 2 clients in one day or 6 in a week. Wow! How things have changed. I am very happy with the success of my business and the amount of effort I have put forth to make things happen. In this business you need to be **assertive.**

In order to share a couple of my days with you I needed to look back in my calendar to see what appointments I had scheduled. When reviewing the day's events I had a not so eventful day...

TIME	ACTION	COMMENT
Travel	40 miles	
4:00 P.M	45 min Massage	cancel
5:00 P.M.	30 min. Massage	cancel
5:45 P.M.	30 min. massage	no-show
6:00 P.M.	45 min. work out	
7:00 P.M.	Massage for myself	felt great!
New Day		
2:00 P.M.	30 min. massage	in town
4:00 P.M.	60 min. massage	40 miles a way
5:30 P.M.	60 min. massage	same location
6:30 P.M.	30 min. massage	same location
8:00 P.M.	arrive home	
New Day		
Travel	40 miles	
11:30 A.M.	15 min. chair massage	out of town cancelled
11:45 A.M.	15 min. chair massage	out of town cancelled
	Spent time prospecting for new chair massage business	
3:30 P.M.	60 min massage	same location

TIME	ACTION	COMMENT
New Day		
7:15 A.M.	Leave for first appointment	
8:00 A.M.	30 min. massage	in town
9:00 A.M.	30 min. massage	same location
Travel	20 miles	
11:00 A.M.	45 min. massage	new location
12:00 P.M.	20 min. massage	same location
Travel	25 miles	
1:00 P.M.	30 min. massage	new location
1:45 P.M.	60 min. massage	same location
3:00 P.M.	60 min. massage	same location
5:00 pm	30 min. massage	same location
Travel	20 miles	
6:00 P.M.	30 min. massage	new location

Some days I have an appointment first thing in the morning, while other times are scheduled for later in the evening. I would like to try and keep the appointments as close together as possible, however it is customer based and what works best for my clients. Accommodation is a crucial element, for success in this business. You can at times be too accommodating and that can hurt your business as well. You need to find a happy medium and try to be flexible.

Another part of a typical day includes the administrative work we do as massage therapist. As a massage therapist you will need to take care of: filing, form creation for health history and soap charts, continuing education classes, printing and folding flyers and/or brochures, marketing layouts and prospecting for new clients, ordering of products we use, keeping records of data on the growth of our business, creating invoices for upcoming on-site chair massage sessions. If you run specials for the month or sell products, that preparation takes time as well. The list is endless.

In order to track my business progress I have created many spreadsheets that I use. I have found that updating my spreadsheets on a weekly basis helps keeps me on track. At a glance, I can see where my business has grown, how many miles I have traveled for any given week or day, review the dollars I have spent for a specific month or year-to-date, and see where I need to put forth more effort in a specific region/area or where I need to cut a region/area loose.

Hopefully the above sheds a little light on how your day can go. There will be times when you are booked back to back and have no breathing space. Enjoy the down time for when you're busy-And you will be busy. Use the down time to help your business grow. Remember—**"you are in charge and your success depends on you."**

A thought to ponder:

Be the best you can be;
For you have that one opportunity to show
the client what you are made of.

Business Owner/Independent Contractor Versus Being An Employee

The decision to become a business owner independent contractor versus an employee is not always an easy one. There are many things to consider for all opportunities.

When choosing to become an independent contractor, an enormous amount of responsibility is placed upon the individual. You need to have the qualities of a person who is self driven, motivated, assertive, and organized and has the ability to create structure for himself.

Not only does the above play an important role in the success of your business, but there is also the amount of time and dedication needed to put forth in making your business thrive. Being financially set can bring stability because your earnings are never guaranteed as an independent contractor.

Independent contractors are responsible for all aspects of their business from licensing to laundry, to the ordering of products to the advertisement and marketing strategy. The days can be long and can involve lots of hard work, depending on how successful you want your business to be. The up swing is that you set the rules, determine the price of your services and the hours you choose to work. Take vacation when you want and schedule personal appointments to your liking.

To own and operate your own business requires meeting specific licensing, codes and statutes that need to be met within the city, state, and county in which you reside.

To open your own establishment, a business plan needs to be prepared and presented to your financial institution prior to loans being obtained. Your business plan needs to be very detailed as to how you plan to operate your business, the amount of business you project and how you can support the loan. I would suggest meeting with an advisor in the field to help you have a better understanding of what criteria needs to be met for being a business owner.

Other things to consider: do you hire employees or is the establishment one that you own and operate? Also the location of the establishment plays a key role-are you located in a strip mall or vacant building within a building? Who is responsible for snow removal, lawn care, and facility maintenance? The list goes on.

There are many aspects of being a business owner that need to be reviewed if that is the route you choose to follow. I personally prefer to be an independent contractor. Currently, my businesses are located within an existing establishment. I find that my business is easy to maintain for I am only responsible for myself as an independent contractor.

Being an employee has its benefits. Your work schedule is predetermined and there is stability in pay if you have set hours along with an hourly rate. The laundry is generally taken care of. Your place of employment may offer benefits such as: 401(K), health and dental insurance, and possible vacation pay; however as an independent contractor you are responsible for those items on your own. And as a employee you are still required to maintain all paperwork and other requirements for this type of work (i.e. all continuing education courses etc.).

There is a lot to think about when deciding how to approach the business aspect of being a massage therapist. The decision should be based on what fits your needs.

A thought to ponder:

Follow the footsteps of one who makes things happen.

Mentors—Finding One That Is Right For You

What comes to mind when you hear the word mentor? Is this a person you look up to? Are you thinking of a person who could lend an ear or coach and guide you through some tough or not so tough decisions? Is there a certain someone you would consider to be a mentor? Is there a certain someone who you respect and whose opinion you value enough to consider them to be a mentor?

We all have that certain someone who we look to for guidance or advice; someone who knows us better than we know ourselves. For me it's Mom and Dad, Thomas, Catherine, Jack, Patti, and Laurie. This is a person we trust with our feelings who won't judge us based on our beliefs, but rather coach and guides us through situations that we feel we need assistance with. I even have a mentor who assists in reviewing my written work and she is awesome. Thanks Laurie!

A mentor views situations from the outside versus the driver seat. A mentor can coach and guide you through different situations or experiences where they may have some personal experience.

I have found a few mentors along the way in my career. I have looked for professionals who not only believe in me as a person, and the abilities that I possess, but who will also be honest with me and tell me what I **need** to hear versus what I **want** to hear.

A mentor can be a great resource in helping you grow and develop your professional skills so you can become the person you want to be.

A thought to ponder:

Beware of your surroundings.

The Importance of Maintaining Client Confidentiality

When speaking of confidentiality, what is your first thought? Do you think about respect, morals, values, and the right to information that has been shared with you in confidence? Do you think about the first time you shared something private and it was shared with others or how you shared someone else's information without thinking about the impact it could have?

As you enter the field of massage therapy, client confidentiality is a concern. Trust, respect and the moral issue of keeping pertinent information to yourself and defining when and where it is appropriate to share such information are all important things to consider.

In the field of massage therapy, confidentiality is more than words shared in a conversation during the massage session. Confidentiality is tied to the information written on the Health History Forms and the Soap Charts. Confidentiality is necessary for any conversation between the therapist and the client in the session. The information based on how the person responds to the session, the clients' personal information about themselves and the information you receive is very personal, and should remain between you and the client.

How do you think your clients would feel if you shared their most inner thoughts and feelings with the next person who steps into your office? The confidentiality between the client and the therapist is crucial in any business setting.

Any time you enter a session with a client (whether they are an existing client or a new one), the level of respect you have for his/her privacy should be your top priority. Remember the time you share with your client is not your time but his or hers.

A thought to ponder:

Body, Mind and Spirit.

Finding Balance Within

Once in awhile WE all need a little 'balance' within, including YOU as a massage therapist. It's pretty hard to convince your clients they need a massage to restore balance and wellness if you do not take the time for a massage yourself.

Working as a massage therapist is a very giving job. You need to reward yourself as well. You will be a better therapist if you take the time to clear your mind and renew your spirit. As you know, a massage is a great way to achieve this.

Also make sure you allow yourself some down time in between appointments for the regrouping and clearing of your mind. Your clients can sense if you are uptight or have a lot going on internally. Take a walk, have a snack or meditate to help yourself regroup. These are all important in achieving balance and wellness within.

If your job allows vacation time, make sure to use it. Taking a small vacation may be the ticket to also help renew your spirit and refresh your body. Who would not like a vacation now and then?

Finding balance for yourself is just as important as helping others find balance in their day-to-day life.

A thought to ponder:

To Know the Expectation is to be Aware.

Implementing Policies and Procedures

Sometime down the road you will be faced with the decision of implementing policies and procedures in order to hold your clients accountable for their scheduled appointments. This can range from specific hours of operation to the client arriving late or missing appointments, to the use of coupons and gift certificates that either have expired or do not apply to them. Either way, this is not the easiest thing to do.

When and how you approach this difficult dilemma is up to you. If the implementation of a cancellation or late appointment policy is shared with your clients from the start your clients will clearly be aware of your expectations as a massage therapist and business owner.

For example cancellation policy could state that 24 hr. notice is required for all appointments that are not going to be kept. Situations will arise such that the client may become ill, have a sick child or encounter an unexpected circumstance that cannot be helped or they just plain forgot. Be sensitive and use your better judgment.

Next, you need to determine if the client is habitual for not showing or canceling appointments. You can implement a service charge or simply choose to no longer work with that client. Again, be sensitive and use your better judgment.

Should a client arrive late inform him/her nicely that you will need to cut the session short in order to stay on schedule for upcoming appointments. Most clients will understand and not make a fuss about it.

Coupons, on the other hand, can be a sticky situation. For instance, you have decided to offer a coupon for first time clients. One of your regular clients brings in the coupon asking if they can use it. Consider this—is this a loyal client who sees you on a regular basis or someone who comes in once a year because they received a gift certificate and are now looking for a price break? If this is a loyal client, allowing them to use the coupon can be a way to show your gratitude for their continued business and support.

The bottom line is—Your time is valuable. And yes, your clients are key to your success; however, no shows and no calls impede upon other potential business, and will affect your bottom dollar.

Setting specific hours of operation allows clients to know when and where you are available. My clients are aware of the travel I do from location to location. They have, at times, offered to meet at whatever establishment convenient to me to facilitate scheduling their appointment. I do appreciate this greatly. So sharing this information with clients can help you in the long run.

If your clients know your expectation upfront certain circumstances and many other situations that you will be confronted with will be more comfortable for you to address.

978-0-595-38983-4
0-595-38983-X